VEGETARIAN
FOOD FOR THOUGHT

Quotations & Inspirations

BY
GAIL DAVIS

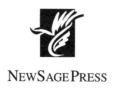

NEWSAGEPRESS

Vegetarian Food for Thought:
Quotations and Inspirations

Copyright ©1999 by Gail B. Davis

Softcover ISBN 0-939165-35-X

NewSage Press
PO Box 607
Troutdale, OR 97060-0607
503-695-2211

web site: http://www.teleport.com/~newsage
email: newsage@teleport.com

Book Design by Nancy L. Doerrfeld-Smith
Illustrations by Sylvia Walker
Cover painting by Patricia Morgan

Printed in the United States on recycled paper with soy ink.

Distributed in the United States and Canada by
Publishers Group West 800-788-2123

Library of Congress Cataloging-in-Publication Data

Davis, Gail (Gail Barbara)
    Vegetarian food for thought : quotations and inspirations / by Gail B. Davis.
        p.   cm.
    Includes bibliographical references.
    ISBN 0-939165-36-8 (alk. paper)
    1. Vegetarianism Quotations, maxims, etc.   I. title.
TX392.D29   1999
613.2'62--dc21
                                                                    99-14519
                                                                         CIP

1   2   3   4   5   6   7   8   9   10

$\mathcal{D}$edicated to the voices of reason.

$\mathcal{I}$NTRODUCTION

Inspiring words can be a gift for any one seeking a more compassionate lifestyle, particularly when feeling alone in his or her beliefs and efforts. I spent three years searching the literature for words of inspiration from others whose lives as vegetarians mirrored my own. The words of conviction, compassion, and courage that I found from vegetarians down through the ages reaffirmed my commitment to embrace a gentler, kinder, and more peaceful way of life. Within these pages you will find many of those inspirational quotations as well as some surprising words of wisdom from the unlikeliest of sources.

I was greatly comforted to learn that there have always been human beings who had the grace and fortitude to speak out on behalf of all living beings. In turn, may their powerful words offer you courage and comfort in your own life as you seek more compassionate ways to eat and live in the world.

VEGETARIAN
FOOD FOR THOUGHT

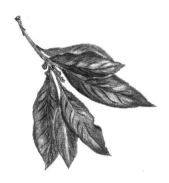

*E*ating vegetables and tofu will keep you in peace.

CHINESE FOLK SAYING

...*E*arth is generous

With her provision, and her sustenance

Is very kind; she offers, for your table,

Food that requires no bloodshed and no slaughter.

OVID BC-17 AD
Roman poet

The Sending of the Animals

The Animals, you say, were "sent"
For man's free use and nutriment.
Pray, then, inform me, and be candid,
Why came they aeons before Man did,
To spend long centuries on earth
Awaiting their Devourer's birth?
Those ill-timed chattels, sent from Heaven,
Were, sure, the maddest gift e'er given —
"Sent" for man's use (can man believe it?)
When there was no man to receive it!

HENRY SALT 1851-1939
Essayist, poet, humanitarian reformer

The average age [longevity] of a meat-eater is 63.

I am on the verge of 85 and still work as hard as ever.

I have lived quite long enough and I am trying to die;

but I simply cannot do it. A single beef-steak would finish me;

but I cannot bring myself to swallow it.

I am oppressed with a dread of living forever.

That is the only disadvantage of vegetarianism.

GEORGE BERNARD SHAW 1856-1950
Dramatist, critic, and social reformer

Non-violence begins at breakfast with what we eat.

INGRID NEWKIRK
Author, activist, co-founder of
People for the Ethical Treatment of Animals

I never liked killing pigs. I never did.
And after "Babe," I absolutely refuse to eat a pig.

OPRAH WINFREY
Talk show host and actress

*I*f you can't conceive of beating an animal,
you shouldn't conceive of eating an animal.

NATALIE MERCHANT
Singer, songwriter

*T*o take away the life of any happy being, to commit acts of depredation
and outrage, and to abandon every refined feeling and sensibility,
is to degrade the human kind beneath its professed dignity of character;
but to devour or eat any animal is an additional violation of those principles,
because it is the extreme of brutal ferocity.

GEORGE NICHOLSON 1760-1825
Author, publisher

Milk is a maternal lactating secretion, a short term nutrient for newborns.
Nothing more, nothing less.

ROBERT M, KRADJIAN, MD

Milk was destined to feed the animal's offspring
and not that man should take it with force for himself.
The kid has the right to enjoy its mother's milk and its mother's love,
but hard-hearted man, influenced by his materialistic and shallow
outlook changes and perverts these true functions.
Thus the gentle kid is unable to partake of its mother's love
and rejoice in the splendor of life.

RABBI ABRAHAM KOOK 1865-1935
First Ashkenazi Chief Rabbi of Israel

There is no biological need for milk.

SUZANNE R. HAVALA, MS, RD

"Milk Has Something for Everybody." Who can argue with that?
Of course that 'something' might be diarrhea, iron-deficiency
anemia, or even a heart attack.

FRANK A. OSKI, MD 1932-1996

If slaughterhouses had glass walls, everyone would be vegetarian.

We feel better about ourselves and better about the animals,

knowing we're not contributing to their pain.

PAUL MCCARTNEY AND
LINDA MCCARTNEY 1942-1998
Musicians

Raise a vegetarian kid for ten years and then give him a bite of steak.
He'll spew it on the ceiling.

BERKELEY BREATHED
Cartoonist

It is only man, mischievous man, that can make death a sport.
Nature taught your stomach to crave nothing but vegetables; but your
violent fondness to change, and greater eagerness after novelties,
have prompted you to the destruction of animals without justice or necessity,
perverted your nature and warped your appetites which way soever
your pride or luxury have called them.

BERNARD DE MANDEVILLE 1670-1733
Physician, satirist

One man is proud when he has caught a poor hare,

and another when he has taken a little fish in a net,

and another when he has taken wild boars,

and another when he has taken bears...Are not these robbers?

MARCUS AURELIUS (ANTONINUS) 121-180 AD
Roman emperor and philosopher

The very people who shudder most over the cruelty of the hunter are

apt to forget that slaughter, in the grimmest sense of the word, is a process they

entrust daily to the butcher and that unlike the game of the forests,

even the dumbest creatures in the slaughterhouse know what

lies in store for them.

LEWIS MUMFORD 1895-1990
Author, social scientist, architect

As we talked of freedom and justice one day for all, we sat down to steaks.
I am eating misery, I thought, as I took the first bite.
And spit it out.

ALICE WALKER
Author

Even if you take animals to be butchered at a remote slaughter house
hundreds of miles away, I believe that all of the animals within a certain radius
can sense that their fellow animals are being slaughtered and they cry
and they may moan because of it. That is why meat can never
be a healthy food: it is pain-poisoned.

SWAMI SATCHIDANANDA
Spiritual leader, author, founder of the Integral Yoga Institute

*A*nimals are my friends...and I don't eat my friends.

GEORGE BERNARD SHAW 1856-1950
Dramatist, critic, and social reformer

I had been thinking about life and relationships
and it dawned on me that my pets were my friends.
I realized then that I could never eat animals.

DARYL HANNAH
Actress

*B*y ceasing to rear and kill animals for food, we can make so much extra food available for humans, that, properly distributed, it would eliminate starvation and malnutrition from this planet.

PETER SINGER
Author, philosopher

The cannibal goes out and hunts, pursues, and kills another man and proceeds to cook and eat him precisely as he would any other game. There is not a single argument nor a single fact that can be offered in favour of flesh eating that cannot be offered, with equal strength, in favour of cannibalism.

DR. HERBERT SHELTON 1895-1985
Naturopathic physician

I never eat anything that comes when you call.

BOBCAT GOLDTHWAIT
Comedian

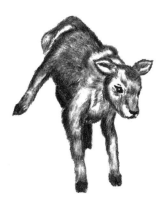

If it has eyes or runs away, don't eat it.

WILL KEITH KELLOGG 1860-1951
Businessman, founder of Kelloggs breakfast cereal company

How good it is to be well-fed, healthy, and kind all at the same time.

HENRY HEIMLICH, MD

Compassion is the foundation of everything positive, everything good.
If you carry the power of compassion to the marketplace and the
dinner table, you can make your life really count.

RUE MCCLANAHAN
Actress

$\mathscr{I}$ think there will come a time, and this is down the road a great
many years, when civilized people will look back in horror on our
generation and the ones that have preceded it: the idea that we should
eat other living things running around on four legs, that we should raise
them just for the purpose of killing them! The people of the future will say,
"meat-eaters!" in disgust and regard us in the same way that we
regard cannibals and cannibalism.

DENNIS WEAVER
Actor

You put a baby in a crib with an apple and a rabbit.
If it eats the rabbit and plays with the apple, I'll buy you a new car!

HARVEY DIAMOND
Author

Certainly man by nature was never made to be a carnivorous animal,
nor is he armed at all for prey and rapine, with jagged and pointed teeth and
crooked claws sharpened to rend and tear, but with gentle hands to gather fruit
and vegetables, and with teeth to chew and eat them.

JOHN RAY 1627-1705
Founder of English Botanical and Zoological Science

The gods created certain kinds of beings to replenish our bodies...

they are the trees and the plants and the seeds...

PLATO 427 BC-347 BC
Greek philosopher

A man can live and be healthy without killing animals for food; therefore,

if he eats meat, he participates in taking animal life merely for the sake

of his appetite. And to act so is immoral.

LEO TOLSTOY 1828-1910
Novelist, moral philosopher, playwright and essayist

$\mathcal{I}$ like the variety of a meatless diet. "What variety?" meat eaters might ask. There are many more varieties of vegetables than there are of meats.

FRED "MISTER" ROGERS

$\mathcal{T}$hose who eat flesh are but eating grains and vegetables at second hand; for the animal receives from these things the nutrition that produces growth. The life that was in the grains and the vegetables passes into the eater. We receive it by eating the flesh of the animal. How much better to get it direct by eating the food that God provided for our use!

ELLEN WHITE 1827-1915
Co-founder of the Seventh Day Adventist Church

*A*nimal factories are one more sign of the extent to which our
technological capacities have advanced faster than our ethics.
We plow under habitats of other animals to grow hybrid corn that fattens
our genetically engineered animals for slaughter. We make free species
extinct and domestic species into biomachines.
We build cruelty into our diet.

JIM MASON AND PETER SINGER
Authors

*I*nsecticides, pesticides, products that are used in paint and preservation of wood, hormones, and animal drugs all turn up in meat.

CAROL TUCKER FOREMAN
Former Assistant Secretary of Agriculture

*B*ased on my experience in Los Angeles, my advice to the public is not to eat meat.

GREGORIO NATAVIDAD
Los Angeles meat inspector for 23 years
in an affidavit filed during an investigation into inspection practices

The foul stream of cruelty must be stopped at its source; the fountain and origin of the evil — the Slaughter-House itself — must be abolished.

HOWARD WILLIAMS 1837-1931
Scholar, author, founder of the Humanitarian League

I think all the social evils can be traced back to the slaughterhouse.
Terrorism. It's only natural we have terrorism.
We've been terrorizing innocents for years, and it's only the karmic
reaction that we start to reap what we sow.

CHRYSSIE HYNDE
Singer, the Pretenders

If we live in peace and love,
we will not kill our fellow creatures for any reason,
even to obtain food.
There is no need to do so when other foods
are available to us that are both healthful and delicious.

PETER MAX
Artist

For my part I have never been able to see, without displeasure,
an innocent and defenseless animal, from whom we receive
no offense or harm, pursued and slaughtered.

MICHEL EYQUEM DE MONTAIGNE 1533-1592
Essayist

If you knew how meat was made, you'd probably lose your lunch.

k.d. lang
Singer, songwriter

I do not see any reason why animals should be slaughtered
to serve as human diet when there are so many substitutes.
After all, man can live without meat.

HIS HOLINESS THE XIV DALAI LAMA

You don't have to give antibiotics to broccoli.

MICHAEL KLAPER, MD

You never hear anybody talk about mad tofu disease.

JOHN ROBBINS
Author, Founder of EarthSave, International

With people in general the very look and touch of raw flesh excite a disgust which only a special education can overcome...The true carnivora and ominivora have no horror of dead bodies; the sight of blood, the smell of raw flesh, inspires them with no manner of disgust. If all of us, men and women alike, were compelled to dispense with the offices of a paid slaughterer and to immolate our victims with our own hands, the penchant for flesh would not long survive in polite society.

DR. ANNA KINGSFORD 1846-1888
Physician and author

I have often thought, if it was not for this tyranny which Custom usurps over us, that men of any tolerable good nature could never be reconciled to the killing of so many animals for their daily food, as long as the bountiful Earth so splendidly provides them with varieties of vegetable dainties.

BERNARD DE MANDEVILLE 1670-1733
Physician, satirist

The longer I don't eat meat, the more dreadful the whole prospect of eating meat is to me. The sight of a butcher shop and slabs of dead animals hanging in the window appalls me. It's a monstrous and uncivilized way of eating.

HAYLEY MILLS
Actress

The most dangerous weapon in the arsenal of the Homo sapiens
is the table fork.

HOWARD LYMAN
Author, Ex-fourth generation cattle rancher

I suggest that in proportion as man is truly "humanized," not by schools
of cookery but by schools of thought, he will abandon the barbarous habit of his
flesh-eating ancestors, and will make gradual progress towards a purer, simpler,
more humane, and therefore more civilized diet-system.

HENRY SALT 1851-1939
Essayist, poet, humanitarian reformer

Go to the meat market of a Saturday night, and see the crowds of
live bipeds staring up at the long rows of dead quadrupeds.
Does not that sight take a tooth out of the cannibal's jaw? Cannibals?
Who is not a cannibal? I tell you it will be more tolerable for the Fejee that
salted down a lean missionary in his cellar against a coming famine —
it will be more tolerable for that provident Fejee, I say, in the day of
judgment, than for thee, civilised and enlightened gourmand, who nailest
geese to the ground and feastest on their bloated livers
in thy pâté de foie gras.

HERMAN MELVILLE 1819-1891
Novelist

COSTELLO: *Do* I have to milk a bunch of cows?

ABBOTT: No. Not bunch, herd.

COSTELLO: Heard what?

ABBOTT: Herd of cows.

COSTELLO: Sure I heard of cows. What do you think I am? A dummy?

ABBOTT: No. A cow herd.

COSTELLO: What do I care if a cow heard? I didn't say anything to be ashamed of.

ABBOTT: Look, please. Do you know what a cow gives? A cow gives milk.

COSTELLO: No she don't. You have to take it away from her.

WILLOUGHBY (LOU COSTELLO) AND DUKE (BUD ABBOTT)
as they are sent to milk cows in the movie
Ride'Em Cowboy (1942)

$\mathscr{I}$ don't myself believe that even when we fulfill our minimum
obligation not to cause pain, we have the right to kill animals.
I know I would not have the right to kill you, however painlessly,
just because I liked your flavour, and I am not in a position to judge
that your life is worth more to you than the animal's to it.

BRIGID BROPHY 1929-1995
Novelist, critic, biographer, philosopher

To my mind, the life of a lamb is no less precious
than that of a human being.
I should be unwilling to take the life of a lamb
for the sake of the human body.

MOHANDAS (MAHATMA) GANDHI 1869-1948

My food is not that of men;
I do not destroy the lamb and the kid
to glut my appetite; acorns and berries
afford me sufficient nourishment.
My companion will be of the same nature as myself,
and will be content with the same fare.

MARY WOLLSTONECROFT SHELLEY 1797-1851
Author, From the book Frankenstein

When Autumn dews filled my eastern garden,
Mustard was so green Turnip so golden,
Which I usually ate with pleasure,
Wondering why men take to eating flesh!

SU TUNG P'O 1036-1101
Chinese poet

The natural sentiments and sympathies of human beings, in regard to
the killing of other animals, are generally so averse to the practice, that few
men or women could devour the animals which they might be obliged
themselves to kill; yet they forget, or affect to forget, the living
endearments or dying sufferings of the creature, while they
are wantoning over his remains.

SIR RICHARD PHILLIPS 1767-1840
Author, publisher, High Sheriff of Middlesex

Animals are not edibles.

HENRY SPIRA 1927-1998
Founder and president of Animal Rights International
and the Coalition for Nonviolent Food

It seems disingenuous for the intellectual elite of the first world
to dwell on the subject of too many babies being born in the second- and
third-world nations while virtually ignoring the over population of cattle
and the realities of a food chain that robs the poor of sustenance to feed
the rich a steady diet of grain-fed meat.

JEREMY RIFKIN
Author, founder of the Pure Food Campaign

A vegetarian diet is one of the most important investments you
can make in yourself and for the world at large.

ANDREAS CAHLING
IFBB Professional Bodybuilder, Mr. International

My refusing to eat flesh occasioned an inconveniency, and I was
frequently chided for my singularity, but, with this lighter repast,
I made the greater progress, from greater clearness of head
and quicker comprehension.

BENJAMIN FRANKLIN 1706-1790
Statesman, author, and inventor

Fruits, nuts, cereal, and vegetation were the basis of the human diet over the millennia. Our modern diet is really an anathema to our whole historical evolution.

OLIVER ALABASTER, MD
Director of the Institute for Disease Prevention,
George Washington University

Comparative anatomy proves that man is naturally a frugivorous animal, formed to subsist upon fruits, seeds, and farinaceous vegetables.

SYLVESTER GRAHAM 1794-1851
Health reformer, author, Presbyterian minister,
inventor of the Graham Cracker

The best use of research money would be to help our society make the transition to a plant-based diet. God has already given us designer foods. They're called grains, beans, and vegetables.

MARK MESSINA, PHD
Author

Why cause suffering to these inferior and innocent orders of being and why take the life that only the gods could give; and why eat flesh, yet dripping with innocent blood? Do not the oracles condemn it? Do they not advise lentils, and grains and fruits that ripen in the sun?

HERODOTUS
C. 5th CENTURY BC
Greek Historian

If we are reasonably sure of what our data from these studies
are telling us, then why must we be reticent about recommending
a diet which we know is safe and healthy?
We, as scientists, can no longer take the attitude
that the public cannot benefit from information they are not ready for.
We must have the integrity to tell them the truth
and let them decide what to do with it.
We cannot force them to follow the guidelines
we recommend, but we can give them these guidelines
and then let them decide.
I personally have great faith in the public.
We must tell them that a diet of roots, stems, seeds, flowers,
fruit, and leaves is the healthiest diet and the only diet we can
promote, endorse, and recommend.

T. COLIN CAMPBELL, PHD
Director, China Health Study

𝒯considered that life was sweet in all living creatures, and taking it away became a very tender point with me...I believe my dear Master has been pleased to try my faith and obedience by teaching me that I ought no longer to partake of anything that had life.

JOSHUA EVANS 1731-1798
Quaker prophet

𝒩o matter what peculiar body a chicken or fish may come in, behind those eyes is a living, feeling being just like me.

INGRID NEWKIRK
Author, activist, co-founder of
People for the Ethical Treatment of Animals

Do we have the right to rear animals in order to kill them
so that we may feed appetites in which we have been artificially
conditioned from childhood?

ASHLEY MONTAGU
Anthropologist and educator

The custom of tormenting and killing of beasts will, by degrees,
harden their hearts even towards men. And, they who delight in the
suffering and destruction of inferior creatures, will not be apt to be very
compassionate or benign to those of their own kind. Children should from
the beginning be brought up in abhorrence of killing or
tormenting any living creature.

JOHN LOCKE 1632-1704
Philosopher

There are a lot of people who believe that in becoming
vegetarian something is missing from your life.
All that's missing is the killing.

EDDY GRANT
Singer, Musician

I have retained her firm belief, that to kill animals for the purpose
of feeding on their flesh is one of the most deplorable and shameful
infirmities of the human state; that it is one of those curses cast
upon man either by his fall, or by the obduracy
of his own perversity.

ALPHONSE LAMARTINE 1790-1869
Poet, historian, statesman
Speaking of his mother in *Les Confidences*

I am against killing and cruelty.

That's why I'll always be a tofu and potatoes man.

KEVIN NEALON
Actor, Comedian

*L*ife remains immoral or only falsely moral, if there is cruelty

and killing for the satisfaction of our daily needs.

SWAMI AVYAKTANANDA 1901-1990
Spiritual teacher and writer, leader of the Vedanta
Movement in Great Britain

World peace, or any other kind of peace, depends greatly on the attitude of the mind. Vegetarianism can bring about the right mental attitude for peace. In this world of lusts and hatreds, greed and anger, force and violence, vegetarianism holds forth a way of life, which if practiced universally, can lead to a better, juster, and more peaceful community of nations.

U NU (THAKIN NU) 1907-1995
Former Prime Minister of Burma

The most important part of vegetarianism is the real shift in consciousness that takes place. There is a true correlation between our food choices and violence in the world. The only person who would disagree with that is a meat-eater.

PETER BURWASH
Tennis professional,
Davis Cup Winner

*L*obsters roasted alive, Pigs whipt to death, Fowls sewed up, are testimonies of our outrageous Luxury. Those who (as Seneca expresses it) divide their lives betwixt an anxious Conscience and a Nauseated Stomach, have a just reward of their gluttony in the diseases it brings with it.

ALEXANDER POPE 1688-1744
Poet

*B*ut to deliver animals to be slaughtered and cooked, and thus be filled with murder, not for the sake of nutriment and satisfying the wants of nature, but making pleasure and gluttony the end of such conduct is transcendently iniquitous and dire!

PORPHYRY 233 AD-304 AD
Greek Neoplatonist. Student and biographer of Plotinus and Pythagoras

I have no doubt that it is a part of the destiny of the human race in its gradual improvement, to leave off eating animals as surely as the savage tribes have left off eating each other when they came into contact with the more civilized.

HENRY DAVID THOREAU 1817-1862
Essayist, naturalist, poet

When I learned what foie gras is and how it's extracted,
I sat down and wept.

BEATRICE ARTHUR
Actress

The unidentifiable slab of meat beneath a cellophane wrapper
is far removed in appearance from its original source.
Thoughtlessly, we often choose not to recognize that it is
the body part of a once living, feeling being.
But, at the deepest spiritual level, each one of us knows that killing is wrong.
That is why there can be no moral or rational justification
for the continual torture and slaughter of billions of sentient beings.

GAIL DAVIS
Author

There can be no purity whilst the flesh of creatures
is partaken of and inhumanity towards the creatures is practiced

RUTH HARRISON
Author

To a man whose mind is free there is something even more intolerable
in the sufferings of animals than in the sufferings of man. For with the latter
it is at least admitted that suffering is evil and that the man who causes it is a
criminal. But thousands of animals are uselessly butchered every day
without a shadow of remorse. If any man were to refer to it, he would
be thought ridiculous. And that is the unpardonable crime.

ROMAIN ROLLAND 1866-1944
Novelist, 1915 Nobel prize laureate

A dead cow or sheep lying in a pasture is recognized as carrion.
The same sort of carcass dressed and hung up in a butcher's stall passes
as food. Careful microscopic examination may show little or no difference
between the fence corner carcass and the butcher's shop carcass.
Both are swarming with colon germs and redolent with putrefaction.

JOHN HARVEY KELLOGG, MD 1852-1943
Surgeon, inventor, and founder of Battle Creek Sanatorium

B iochemically, when a frightened animal knows it's going to be killed,
a rush of adrenalin pulses through its body. After the kill, rigor mortis sets in,
gases form, rot and putrefaction begin, and parasites have a feeding frenzy.
Next, it can be found on someone's dinner plate — yummy!

SPICE WILLIAMS
Actress, stuntwoman, bodybuilder

In their relations with animals, humans eat, hunt, trap, ride, brand, wear, cage, own, sell, breed, dissect, exploit, tame, capture, torture, sacrifice and kill them. This is for starters...Much of this gore and suffering is legal...Much of it is also out of sight, with the meat-aisle shopper or the hamburger-chomper unaware of the pain inflicted on animals in factory farms and slaughterhouses. The human-caused violence done to animals has been normalized, either through habit or culture, so that it's only the oddball who tries to see life also from the animals's viewpoint who is considered abnormal.

COLMAN MCCARTHY
Staff writer for *The Washington Post*

Sacrifices were invented by men as a pretext for eating flesh.

CLEMENT OF ALEXANDRIA (TITUS FLAVIUS CLEMENS) C.150-220 AD
Greek Christian theologian and writer

It is cruel folly to offer up to ostentation so many lives of creatures,

as to make up the state of our treats.

WILLIAM PENN 1644-1718
English Quaker, founder of Pennsylvania

*P*igs and cows and chickens and people are all competing for grain.

MARGARET MEAD 1901-1978
Anthropologist

*N*o single activity or combination of activities has contributed
more to the deterioration of plant and animal life than the nibbling
mouths and pounding hooves of livestock.

RICHARD AND JACOB RABKIN
Naturalists, authors

In my view, no chemical carcinogen is nearly so important
in causing human cancer as animal protein.

T. COLIN CAMPBELL, PHD
Director, The China Health Project

Epidemiological evidence points to the beneficial effects
of a vegan diet in almost every chronic disease.

GEORGE EISMAN, RD
Founder of VEGEDINE, Association of Vegetarian Dieticians and Nutrition Educators

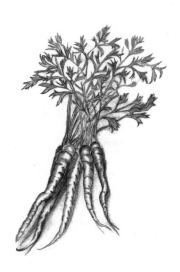

When we eat vegetarian food,

we don't have to worry about

what kind of disease the food died of.

This makes a joyful meal!

JOHN HARVEY KELLOGG, MD 1852-1943
Surgeon, inventor, and founder of Battle Creek Sanatorium

You have just dined, and however scrupulously the slaughterhouse
is concealed in the graceful distance of miles, there is complicity.

RALPH WALDO EMERSON 1803-1883
Essayist, philosopher, and poet

The animals die that we may live, they are substitute people...
And we eat them out of cans or otherwise; we are eaters of death.

MARGARET ATWOOD
Novelist

$\mathcal{I}$ don't eat meat, fish, or dairy. . . I do this because I love animals,
and I don't want to eat them or wear them.
I made this choice and I don't miss anything at all about it.

DREW BARRYMORE
Actress

$\mathcal{A}$ll living beings love their life, desire pleasure, and are averse to pain;
they dislike any injury to themselves; everybody is desirous of life,
and to every being, his own life is very dear...
This is the quintessence of wisdom:
not to injure any living being.

LORD MAHAVIRA 599-527 BC
in the Jain scripture, Sutrakritanga

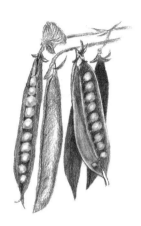

Refrain at all times such foods as cannot be procured without violence and oppression. For know that all the inferior Creatures, when hurt, do cry and send forth their complaints to their Maker.

THOMAS TRYON 1634-1703
Philosopher, author

We must recognize that it is ecological suicide for us to
endeavor to maintain a meat-based agriculture and
a primarily carnivorous diet.

MICHAEL W. FOX
Veterinarian, author

A month ago I became a complete vegetarian.
The moral effect of this way of life — a voluntary subjection of the body
and its ever-increasing demands — is immense. You can understand
how completely convinced I am by it when I tell you that through it
I expect the regeneration of the human race.

GUSTAV MAHLER 1860-1911
Composer, conductor

If animals could talk, would we then dare to kill and eat them?
How could we then justify such fratricide?

FRANCOIS VOLTAIRE 1694-1778
Satirist, philosopher, historian, dramatist, poet

My own personal feeling...is that being a vegetarian makes one
much more pacific as a person. I'm not quite sure whether that's
psychological or whether in fact there is something physiological involved.
But through getting in touch with your inner sea of calm, you also
get in touch with nature and with the beauty
of all aspects of the planet.

ROSE BIRD
Former California Chief Justice

The eating of meat extinguishes the great seed of compassion.

THE BUDDHA (SIDDHARTHA GAUTAMA OR SHAKYAMUNI)
563 BC-483 BC from the The Mahaparinirvana

They tell children, perhaps, that they must not be cruel either
to "Animals" or to human beings weaker than themselves.
But when the child goes into the kitchen, he sees Pigeons, Hens,
and Geese slaughtered and plucked; when he goes into the streets
he sees animals hung up with bodies besmeared with blood, feet cut off,
and heads twisted back...What avails all the fine talk about morality,
in contrast with acts of barbarism and immorality presented to
them on all sides?

GUSTAV STRUVE 1807-1870
Diplomat, writer, humanitarian

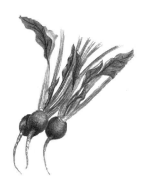

*V*eganism has given me a higher level of awareness and spirituality.

DEXTER SCOTT KING
Son of Martin Luther King, Jr.

I am conscious that flesh eating is not in accordance

with the finer feelings, and I abstain from it.

ALBERT SCHWEITZER, MD, PHD 1875-1965
Philosopher, theologian, Nobel laureate

"Spare Me" Says the Animal

*W*hen a small animal is killed
and trembling, It wants to say "Spare Me" but who is hearing!
I beg all of the mankind who wants peace
Try to have great compassion and stop killing!

MENCIUS C. 380-289 BC
Chinese philosopher

*Y*ou teach children about loving animals — piggies and lambs and cows
and chickens — and then feed them these animals for lunch and for supper.
It seems to me that the process is really in drastic need of overhauling.

CANDICE BERGEN
Actress

You apply the term wild to lions, panthers, and serpents;
yet, in your own savage slaughters, you surpass them in ferocity;
for the blood shed by them is a matter of necessity,
and requisite for their subsistence. But, that man is not,
by nature, destined to devour animal food, is evident...

PLAUTUS C.254-184 BC
Roman dramatist

Human beings are not natural carnivores.
When we kill animals to eat them, they end up killing us
because their flesh, which contains cholesterol and saturated fat,
was never intended for human beings, who are natural herbivores.

WILLIAM C. ROBERTS, M.D.
Editor-in-Chief of the American Journal of Cardiology

$\mathscr{I}$t is incredible how much prejudice has been allowed
to operate in favour of meat, while so many facts are opposed
to the pretended necessity of its use.

PHILIPPE HECQUET, MD 1661-1737
Medical reformer, author

$\mathscr{A}$nd the flesh of slain beasts in his body will become his own tomb.
For I tell you truly, he who kills, kills himself, and who so eats
the flesh of slain beasts, eats the body of death.

THE ESSENE GOSPEL OF PEACE
Direct translation of early Aramaic texts,
recounting the words of Jesus

Vegetable diet and sweet repose. Animal food and nightmare.
Pluck your body from the orchard; do not snatch it from the shambles.
Without flesh diet there could be no bloodshedding war.

LOUISA MAY ALCOTT 1832-1888
Novelist, poet

What with our hooks, snares, nets, and dogs, we are at war with
all living creatures, and nothing comes amiss but that which is either too
cheap or too common; and all this is to gratify a fantastical palate.

SENECA C. 4 BC-65 AD
Roman philosopher and playwright

In my opinion, killing an innocent animal for the temporary luxury
of teasing human taste buds represents grisly and selfishly lopsided logic.
Many eat meat, but few go down to the slaughter house.

ANDY JACOBS, JR.
Former US Representative, D-Indiana

To know that dinner's recipe involved 16 pounds of grain
per pound of beef, enough water to float a battle ship, 150 gallons
of water soaked into the earth flooding it with nitrates,
anywhere from 7 to 24 vaccines and a life of misery ending with
a fearful death and draining its blood, all so someone can burp
at the end of a meal and say "That was good!"
somehow just doesn't seem moral to me.

RIKKI ROCKETT
Musician, drummer for the rock band Poison

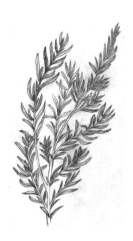

It is only by softening and disguising dead flesh by culinary preparation,
that it is rendered susceptible of mastication or digestion;
and that the sight of its bloody juices and raw horror does not
excite intolerable loathing and disgust.

PERCY BYSSHE SHELLEY 1792-1822
Poet

How dare we pretend to love justice when for the pleasure
of our tongues and palates we murder hundreds of thousands
of defenseless animals in cold blood every day without a 'shadow of remorse'
and without anyone suffering the slightest punishment.
What an evil karma we human beings continue to store up for ourselves,
what a legacy of violence and terror we bequeath future generations!

ROSHI PHILIP KAPLEAU
Zen Master, author

As I cannot kill, I cannot authorize others to kill. Do you see?
If you are buying from a butcher you are authorizing him to kill — to kill
helpless, dumb creatures which neither your nor I could kill ourselves.

PAUL TROUBETZKOY 1866-1938
Sculptor

It is obvious that our natural instinct is not inclined toward flesh food.
Most of us have our meat animals slaughtered for us by proxy, as we would
be sickened if forced to kill these animals ourselves.
Instead of eating meat in its natural state as do all carnivora
and omnivora, we boil, bake, broil or fry it, and usually disguise it
with various gravies and seasonings so that it bears
no real resemblance to the original product.

NATHANIEL ALTMAN
Author

*N*ever be ashamed to say, "No, thank-you; I do not eat meat.

I have conscientious scruples against

eating the flesh of dead animals."

ELLEN WHITE 1827-1915
Co-founder of the Seventh Day Adventist Church

As the trucks rolled by, I saw cows and sheep in those trucks,
being transported. One could only see their eyes through the slits in the trucks,
and it struck me that that was very much like the scene out of the Holocaust
period of Jews being transported in cattle trucks to their fate.
During the Holocaust, I'm sure that the German people were aware
that Jews and others were being treated in the most horrific way.
They may not have known all the details, but they must have known
something, but they didn't want to think about it.
And I think today, we also don't want to think about the way
in which animals are being treated. So there is a parallel in terms
of our desire not to reflect on what is really happening.

RABBI PROFESSOR DAN COHN-SHERBOK
Author, television and radio broadcaster

As often as Herman had witnessed the slaughter of animals
and fish, he always had the same thought: in their behaviour toward
creatures, all men were Nazis. The smugness with which man
could do with other species as he pleased exemplified
the most extreme racist theories, the principle that might is right.

ISAAC BASHEVIS SINGER 1904-1992
Author, Nobel laureate, Holocaust survivor

I don't eat meat because meat brings out negative qualities such as fear, anger, anxiety, aggressiveness, etc. Vegetables peacefully offer themselves to the earth when ripe, thus allowing a sublime and peaceful thought-consciousness.

CARLOS SANTANA
Musician

The indifference of children towards meat is one proof that the taste for meat is unnatural; their preference is for vegetable foods...Beware of changing this natural taste and making children flesh-eaters, if not for their health's sake, for the sake of their character; for how can one explain away the fact that great meat-eaters are usually fiercer and more cruel than other men; this has been recognised at all times and in all places.

JEAN JACQUES ROUSSEAU 1712-1788
Philosopher

*I*t is nothing less than a form of violence to attempt to win children over to the toxic poisons, the coarse flavour and the unsympathetic texture of animal flesh.

JON WYNNE-TYSON
Author

*I*f we don't change our eating habits and go vegetarian,
we cannot continue to feed the world.
Being vegetarian also makes us more humane.
All beings have the right to life.

LINDA BLAIR
Actress

To cause animals to suffer cannot be defended merely on the grounds
that we like the taste of their flesh, and even if animals were raised so that
they lead generally pleasant lives and were 'humanely' slaughtered, that would
not insure their rights, including their right to life, were not violated.

TOM REGAN
Author, philosophy professor

Those cruelties caused by the refinements in cookery are too notorious,
and too often adverted to by different authors, to escape the notice of the public;
and the enormity of the crime of boiling living lobsters and other shell-fish,
and of whipping pigs to death, must be apparent to every one.

LEWIS GOMPERTZ 1784-1861
Inventor, founder of the first organizations
for the prevention of cruelty to animals in England

What have I to do with butchers? Death yawns at me as I walk up
and down this abode of skulls. Murder and blood are written on its stalls.
Cruelty stares at me from the butcher's face. I tread amongst carcasses.
I am in the presence of the slain. The death-set eyes of beasts peer at me and
accuse me...Quartered, disemboweled creatures suspended on hooks plead
with me...I am a replenisher of graveyards. I prowl, amidst other
unclean spirits and voracious demons, for my prey.

AMOS BRONSON ALCOTT 1799-1888
Educator, philosopher, social reformer
Written after shopping for meat for his family

From whence such a hunger in man after unnatural and unlawful food?

Do you dare, O mortal race, to continue to feed on flesh?

Do it not, I beseech you, and give heed to my admonitions.

And when you present to your palates the limbs of slaughtered oxen,

know and feel that you are feeding on the tillers of the ground.

OVID BC-17 AD
Roman poet

$\mathscr{I}$ see shining fish struggling within tight nets, while I hear orioles singing carefree tunes. Even trivial creatures know the difference between freedom and bondage. Sympathy and compassion should be but natural to the human heart.

TU FU 712-770
Chinese poet

$\mathscr{W}$ere it announced tomorrow that anyone who fancied it might, without risk of recriminations, stand at a fourth-story window, dangle out of it a length of string with a meal (labeled 'Free') on the end, wait till a chance passer-by took a bite and then, having entangled his cheek or gullet on the hook hidden in the food, haul him up to the fourth floor and there batter him to death with a knobkerry, I do not think there would be many takers.
Most sane adults would, I imagine, sicken at the mere thought.
Yet sane adults do the equivalent to fish every day.

BRIGID BROPHY 1929-1995
Novelist,critic, biographer, philosopher

$\mathcal{I}$t should not be thought that animals go meekly and willingly into the death chambers — they are filled with terror and resist strongly.

GEOFFREY L. RUDD 1909-1995
Journalist, artist, author

$\mathcal{I}$ do not like eating meat because I have seen lambs and pigs killed. I saw and felt their pain. They felt the approaching death. I left in order not to see their death. I could not bear it. I cried like a child. I ran up a hill and could not breathe. I felt that I was choking. I felt the death of the lamb.

VASLAV NIJINSKY 1890-1950
Ballet dancer and choreographer

I'll predict the winners:

Compassion over cruelty

Healthful eating over harmful gluttony.

MARV LEVY
Former Buffalo Bills head coach

*V*egetarianism serves as the criterion by which we know that

the pursuit of moral perfection on the part of humanity

is genuine and sincere.

LEO TOLSTOY 1828-1910
Novelist, moral philosopher, playwright and essayist

Truly man is the king of beasts for his brutality exceeds theirs.
We live by the deaths of others: we are burial places!

LEONARDO DA VINCI 1452-1519
Artist, scientist, poet, and musician

My decision to be a vegetarian was one of those
fortunate instances where reason and instinct danced together.
Suddenly I couldn't face another piece of cadaver.

LAURA HUXLEY
Author

I began to wonder why we cuddle some animals

and put a fork in others.

HENRY SPIRA 1927-1998
Founder and President of Animal Rights International
and the Coalition for Nonviolent Food

We must be reminded that each morning as dawn breaks,

millions upon millions of animals are slaughtered

for food in town and village the world over: death on production lines,

death en masse, industrial death; they see it,

smell it, they know it is coming.

Neither their sight nor their instincts deceive them.

They know.

BRIGITTE BARDOT
Actress

A vegetarian diet lies at the basis of all reform, whether Civil,
Social, Moral or Religious.

DR. WILLIAM ALCOTT 1789-1859
Author, social reformer, founder of the first American Vegetarian Society

*H*ow far have we the right to take our domination of the animal world?
Have we the right to rob them of all pleasure in life simply to make
more money more quickly out of their carcasses?
Have we the right to treat living creatures solely as
food converting machines? At what point do we acknowledge cruelty?

RUTH HARRISON
Author

We might as well eat the flesh of men as the flesh of other animals.

DIOGENES 400-325 BC
Greek philosopher

Man, then, is not carnivorous but under certain abnormal
conditions; and his senses, to which he appeals in support of his
carnivorousness, are perverted to such a degree, that he would devour
his fellow-man without perceiving it, if they served him up in place
of veal, the flesh of which is said to have the same taste.

JEAN ANTOINE GLEÏZÈS 1773-1843
Philosopher, author

The enlightened mortals of the twentieth century
will surely be vegetarians.

FRANCES WILLARD 1839-1898
Educator, reformer, author

Animals, whom we have once learnt to destroy, without
remorse, we are easily brought, without scruple, to devour.
The corpse of a man differs in nothing from the corpse
of any other animal; and he who finds the last palatable, may,
without much difficulty, accustom his stomach to the first.

JOHN OSWALD 1755-1793
Author

If people could begin to understand that if they could have
respect for all creatures on this Earth, only then can the murdering
of human beings be stopped. But as long as they continue to slaughter
animals, they're going to have wars, and we are not going to find peace.
Peace will come after we discover that we should
have reverence for all living things.

CASEY KASEM
Radio and television personality

Whenever I see a meat and fish-ridden dining table, I know
that I am looking upon one of the seeds of war and hatred —
a seed that develops into an ugly weed of atrocity...
When people ask me,"Is there likely to be a future war?" I answer,
"Yes, until the animals are treated as our younger brothers."

G.S. ARUNDALE 1878-1945
Former President of the Theosophical Society

From cutting the throat of a young calf to cutting the throats
of our brothers and sisters is but a step. While we are ourselves the living
graves of murdered animals, how can we expect any ideal conditions
on the earth?

ISADORA DUNCAN 1878-1927
Pioneer in modern dance

I have from an early age abjured the use of meat,
and the time will come when men such as I will look upon
the murder of animals as they now look upon the murder of men.

LEONARDO DA VINCI 1452-1519
Artist, scientist, poet, and musician

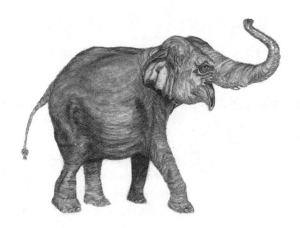

*C*onsider the biggest animals on the planet: elephants, and buffaloes, and giraffes. These are vegetarian animals. They grow to thousands of pounds of muscle and bone without ever eating cheeseburgers or pepperoni pizzas.

MICHAEL KLAPER, MD

*B*ut, for the sake of some little mouthful of flesh
we deprive a soul of the sun and light, and of that proportion
of life and time it had been born to enjoy.

PLUTARCH C.46 AD-120 AD
Greek biographer

*I*n 1968 I became a vegetarian after realizing that animals feel
afraid, cold, hungry, and unhappy like we do.

CESAR CHAVEZ 1927-1993
Labor Union Organizer
National Farm Worker's Association

*W*e consume the carcasses of creatures of like appetites, passions
and organs with our own, and fill the slaughter houses daily
with screams of pain and fear.

ROBERT LOUIS STEVENSON 1850-1894
Novelist, essayist, and poet

*P*eople often say that humans have always eaten animals, as if this
is a justification for continuing the practice. According to this logic,
we should not try to prevent people from murdering other people,
since this has also been done since the earliest of times.

ISAAC BASHEVIS SINGER 1904-1992
Author, Nobel laureate, Holocaust survivor

*U*nder the leadership of Dr. (Martin Luther) King (Jr.) I became totally committed to nonviolence, and I was convinced that nonviolence meant opposition to killing in any form. I felt the commandment 'Thou shalt not kill' applied to human beings not only in their dealings with each other...but in their practice of killing animals for food or sport. Animals and humans suffer and die alike. Violence causes the same pain, the same spilling of blood, the same stench of death, the same arrogant, cruel, and brutal taking of life.

DICK GREGORY
American comedian, author, social reformer, political activist

I publicly apologize for the fact that, for several years,
I was the personification of meat-eating for the Western World.
I sprouted the company line that McDonald's is a happy place.
I didn't tell kids that hamburgers were bad for their health or the
environment. I didn't tell them that hamburger is ground up
dead animals — putrefied rotting flesh on a bun. Instead,
I told them that hamburgers grow in a happy hamburger patch.
For this I am sorry.

GEOFFREY GIULIANO
Former Ronald McDonald actor

The beef industry has contributed to more American deaths than all the wars of this century, all the natural disasters, and all automobile accidents combined. If beef is your idea of "real food for real people," you'd better live real close to a real good hospital.

NEAL BARNARD, M.D.
Author, Director of the Physicians Committee for Responsible Medicine

Meat industry officials have been as aggressive as the bulls of Pamplona in telling America's steak and hamburger lovers to keep chomping away: The carcasses are safe, healthy and every bit as real food for real people as the actor James Garner said in TV commercials they were, before he had a real fine heart bypass operation.

COLMAN MCCARTHY
Staff writer for *The Washington Post*

It should not be believed that all beings exist for the sake
of the existence of man. On the contrary, all the other beings too
have been intended for their own sakes and not for the sake of anything else.

MAIMONIDES (RABBI MOSES BEN MAIMON) 1135-1204
Jewish scholastic philosopher and rabbi

While we ourselves are the living graves of murdered beasts,
how can we expect any ideal conditions on this earth?

GEORGE BERNARD SHAW 1856-1950
Dramatist, critic, and social reformer

The animals of the world exist for their own reasons.

They were not made for humans anymore than black people

were made for whites or women for men.

ALICE WALKER
Author

*E*ach year, the meat-industrial complex abuses and butchers
nearly nine billion cows, pigs, sheep, turkeys, chickens, and other innocent,
feeling animals just for the enjoyment of consumers. Each year, nearly
1.5 million of these consumers are crippled and killed prematurely by heart
failure, cancer, stroke, and other chronic diseases that have been linked
conclusively with the consumption of these animals. Each year, millions
of other animals are abused and sacrificed in a vain search for a
"magic pill" that would vanquish these largely
self-inflicted diseases.

ALEX HERSHAFT, PHD
President, Farm Animal Reform Movement

I don't understand why asking people to eat a well-balanced
vegetarian diet is considered drastic, while it is medically conservative
to cut people open and put them on powerful cholesterol-lowering
drugs for the rest of their lives.

DEAN ORNISH, MD

*E*very 30 seconds on this continent, Canada included,
somebody grabs their chest and falls over with a heart attack.
This is animal fat clogging up the arteries. When you send this material
down to the pathologist and you ask him to analyze it the report always come back
the same. Saturated fat and cholesterol. It's animal fat.
The pathology report never, ever, ever contains the words:
remnants of broccoli, rice, and tofu.

MICHAEL KLAPER, MD

*O*ur survival, as a people and a planet, depends not so much
on our superiority and dominion over nature, but rather in humility
and the willingness to learn what our fellow creatures are trying
to teach us: that all life is sacred and that love is the answer.

JAMES CROMWELL
Actor

*W*hat is nature?...Nature is the solitary tree in the field,
the meadows and the grove; it is that squirrel shyly hiding behind a bough.
Nature is the ant and the bee and all the living things of the earth.
Nature is a river...Nature is all those mountains, snowclad, with the dark blue
valleys and range of hills meeting the sea...One must have a feeling
for all this, not destroy it, not kill for one's pleasure,
not kill animals for one's table.

J. KRISHNAMURTI 1895 - 1986
Philosopher, writer, spiritual teacher

People try to hide the fact that they are actually eating something
that had a face and a heart, someone who had a soul.

PAUL MCCARTNEY
Musician

Some people say, "We believe that animals have no soul."
That is not correct. They believe animals have no soul because
they want to eat the animals, but actually animals do have a soul.

A.C. BHAKTIVEDANTA SWAMI PRABHUPADA
(SRILA PRABHUPADA) 1896-1977
Spiritual leader, Founder-Archarya of the International Society of Krishna Consciousness

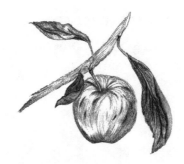

I may look like a man-eater — but I'm actually a vegetarian.

CASSANDRA PETERSON
a.k.a. Elvira Mistress of the Dark

*N*othing will benefit human health and increase chances
for survival of life on Earth as much as the evolution to a vegetarian diet.

ALBERT EINSTEIN 1879-1955
Physicist , Nobel laureate

*T*he issues of cruelty and compassion are obvious in our dietary choices.
What we often fail to recognize is how efficient a vegan diet is. Less land,
less water, more food for our spiraling population.

ED BEGLEY, JR.
Actor, environmentalist

If animals experience not only pain, but also the desire to avoid pain,
why does the meat eater feel justified in causing them unnecessary pain?
Rather than demanding that the vegetarian supply the proof
that a being has rights...perhaps the burden of proof should be
on the meat eater to justify his position in the light
of the pain he causes.

DANIEL A. DOMBROWSKI
Author

A shift to a plant-based diet is one of the most important things, if not the most important thing, that a person can do for people and for our threatened planet.

RICHARD H. SCHWARTZ, PHD
Author and Professor of Mathematics

The argument that a group of individuals is "all alike" has been used throughout human history as a justification for the oppression of that group. If all the individuals are alike, then they become impersonal and killing them seems less wrong or horrendous. Chickens, whether intelligent or stupid, individual or identical, are sentient beings. They feel pain and experience fear. This, in itself, is enough to make it wrong to cause them pain and suffering.

JENNIFER RAYMOND
Author, chef

Animals have taught me so much about love, patience, and beauty —
who could eat the teachers — the angels?

GRACE SLICK
Singer, songwriter

I have been inside abbatoirs; and I can assure you it is terrible
to witness the sufferings of the creatures before they are killed,
and to witness the process by which they are killed, and the effect of such
upon those who kill them. If only men and women could recognize
that the creatures are also little Spiritual
children of the FATHER-MOTHER.

REV. JOHN TODD FERRIER 1855-1943
Christian Leader, Founder of the Order of the Cross

Five tons of poop a piece is just the residue of eating 58 million cattle, 103 million hogs, 300 million turkeys, and nearly nine billion chickens per year, virtually all of whom live and die in conditions that would be prosecutable cruelty if inflicted on a cat, a dog, a horse, or a parrot. Whether you care about animals or just about poop, appropriate action begins with giving up meat.

MERRITT CLIFTON
Animal rights activist

*P*erhaps the most alarming result of our conditioning is the belief that the animals we eat for dinner walk willingly and quietly to a painless and quick death in what is euphemistically termed a "processing plant" to reappear later as a custom-cut main course packed under cellophane at an air-conditioned supermarket, bearing no resemblance whatsoever to the animal from which it originally came.

NATHANIEL ALTMAN
Author

A chop is a piece of leather skillfully attached to a bone
and administered to the patients at restaurants.

AMBROSE BIERCE 1842-1914(?)
Journalist

I'm somewhat shy about the brutal facts of being a carnivore.
I don't like meat to look like animals. I prefer it in the form of sausages,
hamburger and meat loaf, far removed from the living thing.

JOHN UPDIKE
Author

*U*ntil he extends the circle of compassion
to all living things,
man will not himself find peace.

ALBERT SCHWEITZER, MD, PHD 1875-1965
Philosopher, musician, theologian, Nobel laureate

*A*s long as man continues to be the ruthless destroyer
of lower living beings, he will never know health or peace.
For as long as men massacre animals, they will kill each other.
Indeed, he who sows the seeds of murder
and pain cannot reap joy and love.

PYTHAGORAS
6th CENTURY BC
Greek Philosopher and mathematician

*M*an is the only animal that can remain on friendly terms with the victims he intends to eat until he eats them.

SAMUEL BUTLER 1835-1902
Novelist, essayist, and satirist

*M*an has an infinite capacity to rationalize his rapacity, especially when it comes to something he wants to eat.

CLEVELAND AMORY 1917-1998
Journalist, author, Founder-President of the Fund for Animals

*N*ow I can look at you in peace; I don't eat you anymore.

FRANZ KAFKA 1883-1924
Novelist and short story writer
Remark made while admiring fish in an aquarium

*O*ne farmer says to me, "You cannot live on vegetable food solely,
or it furnishes nothing to make bones with," and so he religiously devotes
a part of his day to supplying his system with the raw material of bones;
walking all the while he talks, behind his oxen, which, with vegetable-made
bones, jerk him and his lumbering plow along in spite of every obstacle.

HENRY DAVID THOREAU 1817-1862
Essayist, naturalist, and poet

It was a pleading look,

as if they were asking me not to put them in the pot.

CHEF SIMON BEAVIS,
He quit his job at a seafood restaurant
because he refused to boil lobsters on the grounds of cruelty.

Life! Death! The daily murder, which feeding upon other animals implies —

those hard and bitter problems sternly placed themselves before my mind.

Miserable contradiction! Let us hope that there may be another globe

in which the base, the cruel fatalities of this may be spared to us.

JULES MICHELET 1797-1874
Historian

If a person respects an animal,

how can he suffer it to be killed and eaten?

PIERS ANTHONY
Science fiction writer

And now a third, a Brazen people rise,

Unlike the former, men of monstrous size.

On the crude flesh of beasts, they feed alone,

Savage their nature, and their hearts of stone.

HESIOD
8th CENTURY BC
Greek poet

"*Steak*" just sounds better than carcass.

IMAR HUTCHINS
Author, restaurateur

Dead meat should be buried, not eaten.

CHRISSIE HYNDE
Singer, the Pretenders

In the perfect world originally designed by God,
man was meant to be a vegetarian.

RABBI JACOB COHEN

And God said, Behold, I have given you every herb bearing
seed which is upon the face of the earth, and every tree,
in which is the fruit of a tree yielding seed; to you it shall be for food.

GENESIS 1:29

*Y*ou require flesh if you want to be fat.

MARCUS VALERIUS MARTIAL 43-104 AD
Roman poet

*W*hen your children are adults, and in the prime of their lives,
who's going to tell them that their clogged arteries, malignancies,
and degenerating bodies could so easily have been prevented with
the knowledge you possessed when they were young?

CHARLES ATTWOOD, MD 1932-1998

I refuse to eat animals because I cannot nourish myself by the sufferings
and by the death of other creatures. I refuse to do so,
because I suffered so painfully myself that I can feel the pains of others
by recalling my own sufferings.

EDGAR KUPFER-KOBERWITZ 1906-?
From the essay *Animals My Brethren*
Pages from a secret diary written while a prisoner in Dachau Concentration Camp

How can he be possessed of kindness, who to increase
his own flesh, eats the flesh of creatures?

THIRUVALLUVAR
C. 2nd CENTURY BC
Tamil poet

He who desires to increase the flesh of his own body
by eating the flesh of other creatures
lives in misery...

THE MAHABHARATA
Hindu epic poem

The process of gradual blocking of the coronary arteries
begins not in adulthood but in childhood...and the main cause of this
arteriosclerosis ('hardening of the arteries') is the steadily increasing amount
of fat in the American diet, particularly "saturated" animal fats such as those
found in meat, chicken, milk, and cheeses. If there was another disease
that caused half a million deaths a year, you can be sure that the public
would be acutely aware of the danger, and that the cure
or preventionwould be practiced universally.

BENJAMIN SPOCK, MD 1903-1998

When you see the Golden Arches,
you're probably on the road to the Pearly Gates.

WILLIAM CASTELLI, MD
Director of Framingham Heart Study

The only reason you have a laxative industry
is because you've taken the fiber out of your diet.

DENIS BURKITT, MD 1911-1993

There is no religion without love, and people may talk
as much as they like about their religion, but if it does
not teach them to be good and kind to man and beast,
it is all a sham.

ANNA SEWELL 1820-1878
Author

The assumption that animals are without rights, and the illusion that
our treatment of them has no moral significance, is a positively outrageous
example of Western crudity and barbarity. Universal compassion is
the only guarantee of morality.

ARTHUR SCHOPENHAUER 1788-1860
Philosopher

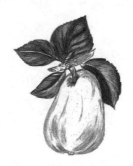

When one becomes a vegetarian it purifies the soul.

ISAAC BASHEVIS SINGER 1904-1992
Author, Nobel laureate, Holocaust survivor

In all the round world of Utopia there is no meat.
There used to be. But now we cannot stand the thought
of slaughter-houses. And in a population that is all educated,
and at about the same level of physical refinement,
it is practically impossible to find anyone who will hew a
dead ox or a pig. We never settled the hygienic question
of meat-eating at all. This other aspect decided us.
I can still remember as a boy the rejoicings over
the closing of the last slaughter-house.

H.G. WELLS 1866-1946
Novelist

Acknowledgements

My deepest appreciation to the many people who contributed so generous-
ly of their time and energy and blessed me with their love and kindness:
Parandeh Amini, Charles Attwood, M.D., Sophia Avants, Menachem Bahir,
Robert Baker, M.D., Neal Barnard, M.D., Ed Begley, Jr., Rynn Berry, Linda
Blair, Patti Breitman, Peter Burwash, Andreas Cahling, Merritt Clifton, Ruth D.
Cookson, Terry Cristofferson, James Cromwell, Edie Davis, Laura Dickterow,
Kit Forage, Alexander Guza, Henry Heimlich, M.D., Alex Hershaft, Laura
Huxley, Stan Jensen, Roberta Kalechovsky, Casey Kasem, Michael Klaper,
M.D., Chiu-Nan Lai, Marv Levy, Howard Lyman, Elena McCaffrey, Colman
McCarthy, John McDougall, M.D., Maureen Michelson, David Morgan,
Patricia Morgan, Israel Mossman, Kannan Nadarajan, Kevin and Linda Nealon,
Jeff and Sabrina Nelson, Ingrid Newkirk, Simon Oswitch, Michael Panarese,
Patricia Rathbone, Jennifer Raymond and Stephen Avis, John and Deo
Robbins, Rikki Rockett, all of the outstanding Santa Barbara Reference
Librarians, Ingrid Sherman, Grace Slick, Nancy L. Doerrfeld-Smith, Terry
Smith, Tania Soussan-Watt and Raymond Watt, Sylvia Walker, Scott Williams,
and Spice Williams and Gregory Crosby.

Akers, Keith, *A Vegetarian Sourcebook*, New York, Putnam, 1983.

Alcott, Louisa May, *Life Letters & Journals*, Grammercy, 1995.

Alcott, William A., *A System of Vegetable Diet,* New York, Fowlers and Wells, 1849.

Altman, Nathaniel, *Eating for Life*, Quest Books, Wheaton, IL, Theosophical Publishing House, 1973.

Attwood, Charles R., *Dr. Attwood's Low-fat Prescription for Kids*, New York, Viking, 1995.

Atwood, Margaret, *Surfacing*, New York, Simon and Schuster, 1972.

Barnard, Neal M.D., *The Power of Your Plate*, Summertown, TN, Book Publishing Company, 1990.

Berman, Louis A., *Vegetarianism and the Jewish Tradition*, New York, KTAV Publishing House, 1982.

Berry, Rynn, *Famous Vegetarians and Their Favorite Recipes*, Los Angeles, Panjandrum Books, 1989.

------------, *The New Vegetarians*, Chestnut Ridge, New York, Townhouse Press, 1988.

Braunstein, Mark Mathew, *Radical Vegetarianism*, Quaker Hill, Connecticut, Panacea Press, 1993.

Brophy, Brigid, *Reads*, London, Sphere Books, 1989.

Bruce, Scott and Crawford, Bill, Cerealizing America: *The Unsweetened Story of American Breakfast Cereal*, Boston, Faber & Faber, 1995.

Butler, Samuel, *The Notebooks of Samuel Butler*, Edited by Henry Festing Jones, Kennerley, 1913.

Cohen, Jacob, *The Royal Table: An Outline of the Dietary Laws of Israel*, 1936, Reprint Jerusalem: Philipp Feldheim, 1970.

Deutsch, Ronald M., *The New Nuts Among the Berries*, Palo Alto, California, Bull, 1977.

Dinshah, H. Jay, *Here's Harmlessness — An Anthology of Ahimsa*, Malaga, New Jersey, American Vegan Society, 1993.

Dombrowski, Daniel A., *The Philosophy of Vegetarianism*, The University of Massachusetts Press, 1984.

Duncan, Isadora, *My Life*, New York, Liveright, 1927.

Ewing, Upton Clary, *The Prophet of the Dead Sea Scrolls*, New York, Philosophical Library, Inc., 1963.

Ferrier, Rev. John Todd, *On Behalf of the Creatures*, London, The Order of the Cross, 1947.

Forget, Carol, *Video Hounds Movie Laughlines: Quips, Quotes & Clever Comebacks,* Gale Research, 1995.

Fox, Michael W., *Inhumane Society*, New York, St. Martin's Press, 1990.

Giehl, Dudley, *Vegetarianism A Way of Life,* New York, Harper & Row, 1979.

Gompertz, Lewis, *Moral Inquiries on the Situation of Man and Brutes*, London, 1924, Reprinted by Centaur Press, Sussex, England, 1992.

Graham, Sylvester, *Lectures on the Science of Human Life,* 2 volumes, Boston, Marsh, Capen, Lyon and Webb, 1839.

Gregory, Dick, *Dick Gregory's Natural Diet for Folks Who Eat: Cookin' with Mother Nature*, New York, HarperCollins, 1974.

Hall, Rebecca, *Voiceless Victims*, Hounslow, Middlesex, Wildwood House, 1984.

Harrison, Ruth, *Animal Machines: The New Factory Farming Industry*, London, Vincent Stuart, 1964.

Hesiod, *Hesiod's Works and Days*, trans. by Walter C. Neale & David W. Tandy, Berkeley, University of California Press, 1996.

Hutchins, Imar, *Delights of the Garden,* New York, Main Street/Doubleday, 1994.

Huxley, Laura Archera, *Between Heaven and Earth*, Santa Monica, Hay House, 1991.

Jarmin, Colin, *Guinness Book of Poisonous Quotes*, Chicago, Contemporary Books, 1993.

Kalechovsky, Roberta, *Rabbis and Vegetarianism: An Evolving Tradition,* Marblehead, Massachusetts, Micah Publications, 1995.

Kapleau, Roshi Philip, *To Cherish All Life: A Buddhist Case for Becoming Vegetarian*, San Francisco, Harper & Row, 1981.

Kellogg, John Harvey, *The Miracle of Life,* Battle Creek, Michigan, Good Health Publishing, 1904.

--------------------, *The Natural Diet of Man*, Battle Creek, Michigan, Modern Medicine, 1923.

Kingsford, Anna, MD, *The Perfect Way in Diet,* London, Kegan Paul, 1881

Mandeville, Bernard de, *Collected Works Vol. III: Fable of the Bees*, George Olms, 1981.

Mason, Jim & Singer, Peter, *Animal Factories,* New York, Harmony, 1990.

Max, Peter & Proust, Ronwen Vathsala, *The Peter Max New Age Organic Vegetarian Cookbook*, New York, Pyramid Books, 1971.

Melville, Herman, *Moby Dick*, London, Richard Bentley, 1851.

Messina, Mark et al., *The Simple Soy Bean & Your Health*, Garden City Park, New York, Avery, 1994.

Messina, Virginia & Messina, Mark, *The Vegetarian Way,* New York, Crown Publishing, 1996.

Najinsky, Waslaw & Najinsky, Romola, *Diary of Vaslav Najinsky,* Berkeley, University of California Press, 1972.

Oski, Frank A., *Don't Drink Your Milk!*, Brushton, New York, Teach Services, 1992.

Oswald, John, *The Cry of Nature*, London, J. Johnson, 1791.

Ovid, *Metomorphoses*, Oxford University Press, 1986.

Peter, Laurence J., *Peter's Quotations: Ideas for Our Time,* New York, William Morrow, 1977.

Phillips, Sir Richard, *Golden Rules of Social Philosophy,* London, J and C Adlard Printers, 1826.

Plutarch, *Moralia*, translated by Harold Cherniss and William Helmbold, Heinemann, 1976.

Pope, Alexander, *The Poems of Alexander Pope,* An Essay on Man: Epistle II, ed. by John Butt, Yale University Press, 1963.

Porphyrius, *Porphyry on Abstienece from Animal Food*, Ed. by Esme Wynne-Tyson, Translated by Thomas Taylor, London, Centaur Press, 1095.

Powell, Horace B., *The Original Has This Signature: W.K. Kellogg*, Englewood Cliffs, New Jersey, Prentice-Hall, 1956.

Rabkin, Richard and Jacob, *Nature in the West,* New York, Holt, Rinehart and Winston, 1982.

Regan, Tom, *All That Dwell Therein*, Berkeley, University of California Press, 1982.

Rifkin, Jeremy, *Beyond Beef:The Rise and Fall of the Cattle Culture*, New York, Dutton, 1992.

Robbins, John, *Diet for a New America*, Walpole, New Hampshire, Stillpoint, 1987.

Rolland, Romain, Jean-Christophe: *Journey's End*, Paris, Albin Michel, 1931.

Rousseau, Jean Jacques, *Emile*, translated by Barbara Foxley, New York, Dutton, 1911.

Rudd, Geoffrey L., *Why Kill for Food?*, Cheshire, England, The Vegetarian Society, 1956.

Salt, Henry, *The Logic of Vegetarianism Essays and Dialogues*, London, George Bell and Sons, 1906.

-----------------, *Animals' Rights: Considered in Relation to Social Progress*, Clarks Summit, Pennsylvania, Society for Animal Rights, 1980.

Schopenhauer, Arthur, *On the Basis of Morality*, Hackett Pub. Co., 1995.

Schweitzer, Albert, *Reverence for Life*, Irvington Pub., 1993.

Seneca, *Moral Essays*, translated by J.W. Basone, Loeb Classical Library, Harvard University Press, 1979.

Sewell, Anna, *Black Beauty,* New York, Macmillan, 1902.

Shelley, Mary Wollstonecroft, *Frankenstein, or The Modern Prometheus: The 1818 Text*, Indianapolis, Bobbs-Merrill, 1974.

Shelley, Percy Bysshe, *A Vindication of Natural Diet*, London, F. Pitman, 1884.

-----------------------------, *On the Vegetable System of Diet*, Ashingdon, Rockford, Essex, London Vegetarian Society by CW Daniel, 1947.

Shelton, Herbert, *Superior Nutrition*, San Antonio, Willow, 1982.

Singer, Peter, *Animal Liberation*, New York, Avon Books, 1977.

Spiegel, Marjorie & Walker, Alice, *The Dreaded Comparison: Human and Animal Slavery*, New York, Mirror Books, 1997.

Szekely, Edmond Bordeaux, *The Essene Gospel of Peace*, Nelson, British Columbia, International Biogenic Society, 1981, 64 pp.

Thoreau, Henry David, *Walden*, Limited Editions Club, 1936.

Tolstoy, Leo, *The First Step*, The Manchester Vegetarian Society, 1902.

-----------------, *Writings on Civil Disobedience and Nonviolence*,

Tryon, Thomas, *The Way to Health, Long Life, and Happiness*, London, 1683.

Vaclavik, Charles P., *The Vegetarianism of Jesus Christ*, Three Rivers, California, Kaweah Publishing, 1986.

Voltaire, Francois, *The Princess of Babylon*.

Wells, H.G., *A Modern Utopia*, London, W. Collins, Sons, & Co., 1905.

White, Ellen G., *Health and Happiness* (originally *Ministry of Healing*, 1905), Phoenix, Inspiration Books, 1973.

-------------------, *Counsels on Diet and Foods*, Tacoma Park, Review and Publishing Association, 1938.

Williams, Howard, *The Ethics of Diet,* London, John Heywood, 1883.

Wynne-Tyson, Jon, *The Extended Circle — A Commonplace Book of Animal Rights*, New York, Paragon House, 1989.

----------------------, *Food for a Future*, New York, Universe Books, 1979

PERIODICALS, LETTERS, and JOURNALS

American Dietetic Association Position Paper on Vegetarian Diets
American Journal of Cardiology, October 1990.
Animal Times, August/September 1994.
------------------, January/February 1995.
Beyond Beef Newsletter, Fall 1993.
"The Decline and Fall of the Meat Industry," Alex Hershaft, Ph.D.
Herald of the Cross, Vol. II, 1906.
International Herald Tribune, April 9, 1996.
J. Krishnamurti Letters to the Schools, Volume 2, 1st November 1983.
Jane, September/October 1997.
"The Milk Letter, A Message to My Patients," Robert M. Kradjian, M.D.
Moneysworth, April, 1979.
Newsweek, March 24, 1997.
MS. magazine, "Am I Blue?", July, 1986
---------------, May 20, 1996.
Nutrition Advocate, December 1995.
-------------------------, January 1996.
PETA News , May/June 1990.
------------------, September/October 1990.
Poultry Press, Fall/Winter 1998.
Seattle Magazine, April 1994.
The Vegetarian, March 1992.

Vegetarian Times, January/February 1981.
----------------------, June 1984.
----------------------, March 1985.
----------------------, September 1985.
----------------------, November 1985.
----------------------, September 1987.
----------------------, May 1988.
----------------------, December 1988.
----------------------, January 1991.
----------------------, October 1995.
The Vegetarian Way, XIX, 1967.
----------------------, XXIV, 1977.
Veggie Singles News, Vol. 6, Spring, 1996.
Vibrant Life, Going Meatless issue, 1992.
The Washington Post, "USDA's Not-So-Meaty Advice," January 9, 1996.

VIDEO & TELEVISION

A Diet for All Reasons, Michael Klaper, M.D. Nutritional Services, 1992.
To Love or Kill: Man vs. Animal, Home Box Office and Carlton UK Television, 1995.

INDEX

Abbott, Bud & Costello, Lou	31	
Alabaster, Oliver, M.D.	37	
Alcott, Amos Bronson	76	
Alcott, Louisa May	65	
Alcott, Dr. William	83	
Altman, Nathaniel	69, 106	
Amory, Cleveland	109	
Anthony, Piers	112	
Arthur, Beatrice	47	
Arundale, G.S.	86	
Attwood, Charles M.D.	115	
Atwood, Margaret	55	
Aurelius, Marcus (Antoninus)	10	
Avyaktananda, Swami	43	
Bardot, Brigitte	82	
Barnard, Neal M.D.	93	
Barrymore, Drew	56	
Beavis, Simon	111	
Begley, Ed Jr.	101	
Bergen, Candice	62	
Bierce, Ambrose	107	
Bird, Rose	59	
Blair, Linda	74	
Breathed, Berkeley	9	
Brophy, Brigid	32, 78	
Buddha (Siddhartha Gautama)	60	
Burkitt, Denis, M.D.	118	
Burwash, Peter	44	
Butler, Samuel	109	
Cahling, Andreas	36	
Campbell, T. Colin Ph.D.	39, 53	

Castelli, William, M.D.	118	
Chavez, Cesar	89	
Chinese Folk Saying	1	
Clement of Alexandria	51	
Clifton, Merritt	105	
Cohen, Rabbi Jacob	114	
Cohn-Sherbok, Dan, Rabbi Professor	71	
Cromwell, James	98	
da Vinci, Leonardo	81, 87	
Davis, Gail	47	
Diamond, Harvey	18	
Diogenes	84	
Dombrowski, Daniel A.	102	
Duncan, Isadora	87	
Einstein, Albert	101	
Eisman, George R.D.	53	
Emerson, Ralph Waldo	55	
The Essene Gospel of Peace	64	
Evans, Joshua	40	
Ferrier, Rev. John Todd Ferrier	104	
Foreman, Carol Tucker	22	
Fox, Michael W.	58	
Franklin, Benjamin	36	
Gandhi, Mohandas	33	
Genesis 1:29	114	
Giuliano, Geoffrey	92	
Gleïzès, Jean Antoine	84	
Goldthwait, Bobcat	15	
Gompertz, Lewis	75	
Graham, Sylvester	37	
Grant, Eddy	42	

Gregory, Dick	91	
Hannah, Daryl	12	
Harrison, Ruth	48, 83	
Havala, Suzanne R. M.S., R.D.	7	
Hecquet, Philippe M.D.	64	
Heimlich, Henry M.D.	16	
Herodotus	38	
Hershaft, Alex Ph.D.	96	
Hesiod	112	
His Holiness the XIV Dalai Lama	25	
Hutchins, Imar	113	
Huxley, Laura	81	
Hynde, Chryssie	23, 113	
Jacobs, Andy Jr.	66	
Kafka, Franz	110	
Kapleau, Roshi Philip	68	
Kasem, Casey	86	
Kellogg, John Harvey M.D.	49, 54	
Kellogg, William Keith	15	
King, Dexter Scott	61	
Kingsford, Dr. Anna	27	
Klaper, Michael M.D.	26, 88, 97,
Kook, Rabbi Abraham	6	
Kradjian, Robert M. M.D.	6	
Krishnamurti, Jiddu	98	
Kupfer-Koberwitz, Edgar	116	
LaMartine, Alphonse	42	
lang, k.d.	25	
Levy, Marv	80	
Locke, John	41	
Lyman, Howard	29	

the Mahabharata	117	Oswald, John	85	Seneca	65
Lord Mahavira	56	Ovid	1, 77	Sewell, Anna	119
Mahler, Gustav	58	Penn, William	51	Shaw, George Bernard	3, 12, 94
Maimonides (Rabbi Moses ben		Peterson, Cassandra	100	Shelley, Mary Wollstonecroft	33
Maimon)	94	Phillips, Sir Richard	34	Shelley, Percy Bysshe	67
Mandeville, Bernard de	9, 28	Plato	19	Shelton, Dr. Herbert	14
Martial, Marcus Valerius	115	Plautus	63	Singer, Isaac Bashevis	72, 90, 120
Mason, Jim	21	Plutarch	89	Singer, Peter	13, 21
Max, Peter	24	Pope, Alexander	45	Slick, Grace	104
McCarthy, Colman	50, 93	Porphyry	45	Spira, Henry	35, 82
McCartney, Linda	8	Prabhupada, A.C. Bhaktivedanta		Spock, Benjamin M.D.	117
McCartney, Paul	8, 99	Swami (Srila Prabhupada)	99	Stevenson, Robert Louis	90
McClanahan, Rue	16	Pythagoras	108	Struve, Gustav	60
Mead, Margaret	52	Rabkin, Richard and Jacob	52	Su Tung P'O	34
Melville, Herman	30	Ray, John	18	Thiruvalluvar	116
Mencius	62	Raymond, Jennifer	103	Thoreau, Henry David	46, 110
Merchant, Natalie	5	Regan, Tom	75	Tolstoy, Leo	19, 80
Messina, Mark Ph.D.	38	Rifkin, Jeremy	35	Troubetzkoy, Paul	69
Michelet, Jules	111	Robbins, John	26	Tryon, Thomas	57
Mills, Hayley	28	Roberts, William C. M.D.	63	Tu Fu	78
Montaigne, Michel Eyquem de	24	Rockett, Rikki	66	Updike, John	107
Montagu, Ashley	41	Rogers, Fred "Mister"	20	Voltaire, Francois	59
Mumford, Lewis	10	Rolland, Romain	48	Walker, Alice	11, 95
Natavidad, Gregorio	22	Rousseau, Jean Jacques	73	Weaver, Dennis	17
Nealon, Kevin	43	Rudd, Geoffrey L.	79	Wells, H.G.	121
Newkirk, Ingrid	4, 40	Salt, Henry	2, 29	White, Ellen	20, 70
Nicholson, George	5	Santana, Carlos	73	Willard, Frances	85
Nijinsky, Vaslav	79	Satchidananda, Swami	11	Williams, Howard	23
U Nu (Thakin Nu)	44	Schopenhauer, Arthur	119	Williams, Spice	49
Ornish, Dean M.D.	97	Schwartz, Richard H. Ph.D.	103	Winfrey, Oprah	4
Oski, Frank, M.D.	7	Schweitzer, Albert MD, Ph.D.	61, 108	Wynne-Tyson, Jon	74

About the Author

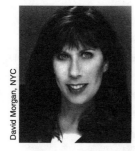

David Morgan, NYC

Gail Davis is a nutritional consultant, speaker and author of *The Complete Guide to Vegetarian Convenience Foods*, (NewSage Press 1999) which is the new and updated version of the original edition, *So, Now What Do I Eat*. Her newspaper column *"Eat your Vegetables!"* appears regularly in the *Albuquerque Weekly Alibi*.

A vegetarian for more than a decade, she has interviewed many prominent physicians, scientists and nutritional experts and written about the relationship between our food choices and their impact on human health.

Davis teamed up with New Jersey physician Robert Baker, and successfully fought for the passage of legislation concerning the prevention of breast cancer. The bill requires doctors in New Jersey to supply patients with a pamphlet describing the connection between diet and breast cancer.

Davis lives in Albuquerque, New Mexico with her feline companion, Indiana Jones, and canine companion, Cicely Alaska, both confirmed vegetarians.

For more information on other books published by NewSage Press:

http://www.teleport.com/~newsage

NEWSAGE PRESS

phone (503) 695-2211
fax (503) 695-5406
email newsage@teleport.com